TEACH YOURSELF ACUPUNCTURE

A Beginner's Guide for the Busy Health Professional

Dr Paul R Weaver

MB, BS (Lond.), Dip. Obst. (Otago), MRNZCGP

Spinal Publications New Zealand Ltd

First published in 1998 by
Spinal Publications New Zealand Ltd
PO Box 93, Waikanae
Wellington, New Zealand
Telephone: ++64 4 293 7020
Fax: ++64 4 293 2897
Email: spinal@xtra.co.nz

ISBN 0-9583647-4-5

Edited by Jan McKenzie and Nada Brajkovich
Printed by Brebner Printing Co. Ltd, Napier, New Zealand

CONTENTS

CHAPTER FOUR

CHAPTER FIVE

INTRODUCTION

Latin definition of acupuncture:
acus—needle *punctura*—penetrate

> Acupuncture is a safe, simple and effective treatment for many of the conditions a health professional will meet in everyday practice. *Teach Yourself Acupuncture* will meet the needs of all those interested in exploring acupuncture as a way of complementing their regular therapies. It is designed to provide the basic information and confidence required to pick up an acupuncture needle and 'get started'. This handbook is suitable for health professionals with a good grounding in anatomy (e.g. doctors, nurses, physiotherapists, chiropractors and osteopaths). I hope that, with encouragement from good results, *Teach Yourself Acupuncture* will whet your appetite for practising and learning more advanced acupuncture. We must, however, acknowledge our own limitations in diagnostic skill by frequently and critically appraising results and considering more serious pathology.

I am a general medical practitioner in New Zealand . My introduction to acupuncture was in 1992 when I attended a course in Australia, taught by Professor Anton Jayasuriya of Sri Lanka. My wife, Michele, wanted a holiday in the sun and despite my initial scepticism persuaded me to do this course, telling me that I would love being an acupuncturist as I seemed to enjoy sticking needles in people.

As it turned out she was right. Anton is a charismatic teacher and immediately inspired me to 'take up the needle'. His textbook, *Clinical Acupuncture*, should be considered compulsory reading for all acupuncturists.

On returning home to Southland I started to practice my new skills on virtually every patient who did not faint or flee at the mention of acupuncture. I was immediately struck by the good results and with time acupuncture has increasingly replaced my standard treatments for many everyday conditions.

The inspiration for this book came in early 1996 from my studies towards the Acupuncture Unit of the Diploma of Family Medicine from Monash University, Victoria, Australia. This is a distance learning programme under the guidance of Dr Geoff Greenbaum. Geoff is also a very inspiring teacher and totally committed to the therapeutic laser as an alternative to needles.

CHAPTER ONE

WHAT IS ACUPUNCTURE USEFUL FOR?

It is particularly good for all musculo-skeletal and painful disorders. These are the areas supported by most of the scientific research into acupuncture. However, a wide range of dysfunctional problems (with no overt pathology or disease process) also respond well.

Some of the conditions with which I have had success include:

- irritable bowel syndrome
- low back pain and pseudosciatica
- pre-menstrual tension
- dysmenorrhoea and endometriosis
- headaches and migraine
- vertigo
- soft tissue injury (sprained ankle)
- trigeminal neuralgia
- tennis and golfer's elbow
- arthritic pain
- dyspepsia
- cholecystitis
- chronic bronchitis
- chronic fatigue
- thrombocytopenia
- eczema, hayfever and asthma
- hyperemesis gravidum
- labour pain
- shoulder dysfunction (e.g. rotator cuff tendonitis)

- costochondritis
- torticollis
- whiplash
- fever
- fibromyalgia and regional pain syndromes
- psoriasis

These conditions can often be difficult to treat with conventional therapy. You can see, therefore, how useful acupuncture could be in expanding your therapeutic approach.

For further information and an overview of acupuncture and its place in current practice read:

Cohen M, 1994, Acupuncture in Australia: a review of its current position, *Journal of the Australian Medical Acupuncture Society*, vol. 12, no. 1, pp. 8–15.

Strauss S, 1987, Acupuncture in perspective, *Australian Family Physician*, vol. 16, no. 1, pp. 39–40.

For a good glossary of acupuncture terms read:

Strauss S, 1987, Glossary of acupuncture terms, *Australian Family Physician*, vol. 16, no. 4, pp. 416–417.

QI (CHI) AND ENERGETIC MEDICINE

The philosophy of traditional Chinese medicine is based around the idea that there is a vital energy of life (chi) which has contrasting and opposite forces (yin and yang). This vital energy flows through the five elements (fire, earth, metal, water and wood) that go to make up all human life forms. The human body can even be considered a microcosm of the greater world, or even universe, which is likewise divided into the five elements. The balance of the energy flow within the elements determines the character of an illness or person.

In health the flow of energy is unhindered and the elements are in a natural balance. In sickness the energy flow is obstructed, leading to excesses and deficiencies of chi and predominance of yin or yang and the different elements. Diagnosis characterises the illness according to these principles and treatment is aimed at returning the normal flow of chi.

Chi flows superficially over the body in meridians (maps and paths), and deeply through the organs. It has a predetermined route, flowing from one meridian and / or organ to the next. There is a predetermined rhythmic time course, with each twenty-four hours comprising one complete cycle (cf. circadian rhythm). This time course starts in the heart meridian. Acupuncture can therefore be used to increase (tonify) energy in a meridian or to reduce (sedate) it.

And so it goes on. If you are baffled at this point don't despair. Remember these theories were invented to explain phenomena observed before 250 BC (when they were first set down in the *Yellow Emperor's Text of Internal Medicine*). There was very little knowledge of the internal workings of the human body at that time. Thus a very complex and flowery set of 'rules' were developed that, while helpful, are not strictly necessary to practice simple acupuncture today.

For further information on the philosophy of traditional Chinese medicine read:

Jayasuriya A, *Clinical Acupuncture*, 11th edn, Medicina Alternativa International, Sri Lanka, pp. 277–328.

Schneideman I, 1988, *Medical Acupuncture: Acupuncture and the Inner Healer*, Mayfair Medical Supplies Ltd, Hong Kong, ch. 8.

Helms J M, 1995, *Acupuncture Energetics: A Clinical Approach for Physicians*, Medical Acupuncture Publishers, Berkeley, California, USA.

Some of the theories are:

1. **Neurological**— gate control theory, thalamic neurone theory etc.

2. **Humeral**— serotonin, endorphins and other neurotransmitters etc.

3. **Bioelectric**— reduced electrical resistance at skin acupuncture points etc.

4. **Placebo Effect**— commonly touted by sceptics

5. **Traditional Chinese Medicine**— modern is a relative term!

6. **Others**— embryological, psychogenic etc.

Most of the research into the mechanism of action of acupuncture has dealt with its analgesic effect. There seems to be clear evidence and good hypothesis that acupuncture analgesia stems from its effects in several layers of the peripheral and central nervous system. Anyone who has inserted an acupuncture needle will have seen the surrounding red ring of histamine release that this can cause in the skin. This demonstrates an ability to alter local chemical and neurotransmitter substances at skin level.

I am sure that there is a segmental reflex action exerted as these impulses reach the spinal cord. This may in part explain the non-analgesic effects of acupuncture, possibly by influence over the autonomic nervous system (see fig. 1).

In 1926, for example, it was discovered that stimulating the epigastrium with temperature changes produced reflex changes in the musculature of the stomach (a cutaneo-visceral reflex).

Again, many of the acupuncture points, especially those on the back, have influence over the internal organs and can be found in the appropriate dermatome, which has segmental connections.

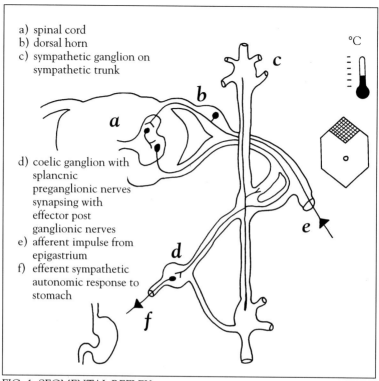

a) spinal cord
b) dorsal horn
c) sympathetic ganglion on
   sympathetic trunk

°C

d) coelic ganglion with
   splancnic
   preganglionic nerves
   synapsing with
   effector post
   ganglionic nerves
e) afferent impulse from
   epigastrium
f) efferent sympathetic
   autonomic response to
   stomach

FIG. 1. SEGMENTAL REFLEX

Pain is recognised by the sensory cortex after travelling a
step-wise route via the spinothalamic tract, through the
spinal cord and thalamus. When the sensation of
acupuncture reaches the spinal cord it sets off a chain
reaction of interference to the transmission of the pain
impulses. Heavily implicated in this are newly-discovered
neurotransmitters called enkephalins, endorphins and
dynorphins, also serotonin and noradrenergic neurones.
They are not exclusive to pain pathways and much of
acupuncture's non-analgesic secrets are yet to be elucidated.

The description of *diffuse noxious inhibitory controls* is compelling. It is a phenomenon whereby a second, potentially noxious stimulus (i.e. acupuncture) can modulate or block the pain sensation of the first. The second stimulus activates the brainstem and descending pathways to block background 'noise' and heighten the clarity of the second painful stimulus. In so doing the original pain is blocked.

Enkephalins are involved as transmitters in the brainstem, and serotonin and noradrenergic neurones in the descending modulatory pathways. This has been termed 'counter irritation'.

Endorphin levels rise after acupuncture, both in the cerebrospinal fluid and the blood stream, and mediate their own opiate type analgesia. This analgesia is mediated at several levels in the pain pathway and arises from the hypothalamus.

Little has yet emerged regarding the mode of action in non-painful medical conditions. Stress causes release of sympathomimetics, adrenocorticotrophic hormone (ACTH), and cortisol. Cortisol would be helpful in some conditions such as atopy or asthma, but that still does not explain the effectiveness of acupuncture. Much research therefore has been done to try to prove the traditional Chinese theories of acupuncture points and meridians. It has to be said that this is less convincing than the research into analgesia. It has been postulated that the electrical skin resistance is reduced at acupuncture points and that these are connected electrically in the form of meridians, with the points acting as voltage generators. There seems to be little good evidence of this, however. Histologically, acupuncture points are no different to ordinary skin, although there may be some merit in the theory that small nerves penetrate the superficial fascia in areas that correspond to acupuncture points (cadaveric observation only).

Anyone doing musculo-skeletal *dry needling* will quickly realise that motor points of muscles, trigger points and acupuncture points are the same thing. So where does that lead us?

Sceptics quote the placebo effect. This is thought to be effective in 30 percent of chronic pain and far less in acute pain. Acupuncture statistics are far better than this with 55 percent to 85 percent success in chronic pain and often similar results in acute pain.

There is much work still to be done if the mechanisms of action of acupuncture are to be elucidated and then hopefully refined. I am sure they will turn out to be multiple and complex.

For further information read:

Man F, 1997, *Scientific Aspects of Acupuncture*, William Heinemann Medical Books Ltd, London, pp. 1–29.

Stux G & Pomeranz B, 1991, *Scientific Bases of Acupuncture*, 2nd edn, Springer-Verlag, New York pp. 4–55.

National Health and Medical Research Council, 1989, *Report of the Working Party on Acupuncture*, Canberra, pp. 1–29.

Strauss S, 1987, The scientific basis of acupuncture, *Australian Family Physician*, vol.16, no.2, pp. 166–169.

Helms J M, 1995, *Acupuncture Energetics: A Clinical Approach for Physicians*, Medical Acupuncture Publishers, Berkeley, USA, ch. 2, pp. 19–69.

CHAPTER TWO

NEEDLES AND NEEDLE STIMULATION (INCLUDING PERIOSTEAL PECKING)

Most medical equipment companies stock acupuncture needles. They are usually boxed in packs of 100 disposable needles. As a beginner, ask for needles with plastic guide tubes. As for size, buy 0.3 x 25mm initially and then you can order longer needles for, say, the buttocks or smaller needles for the face and auriculotherapy later.

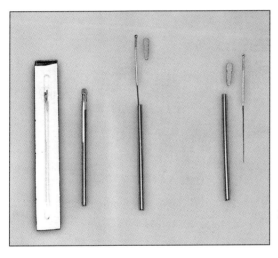

1. Needles with Plastic GuideTubes

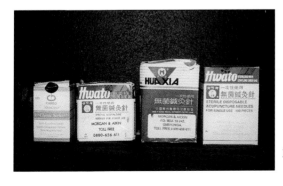

2. Acupunture Needles

It is a good idea to get a catalogue of acupuncture supplies at the start to familiarise yourself with what is available. My personal favourite is the *Hwato* brand with copper handle.

Disposable needles are cheap and protect against cross infection between patients, without the need for an autoclave. In times when AIDS and hepatitis are so prominent, patients often ask me if the needles are disposable.

From packet to skin penetration

Practice this on a willing subject before working with patients: try inserting a needle at LI4 (see also page 28).

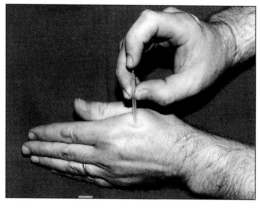

3. Needle Insertion LI4

- Remove the sterile wrapper.
- Some people clean the skin with alcohol but I personally do not feel this is necessary.
- Remove the small tab holding the needle in the guide tube.
- Support the needle handle in the tube with your finger and continue to hide the point.
- Press the needle end of the tube against the skin (this tenses the skin under the needle making insertion less painful).

16

- Tap the top of the needle handle with the index finger of your free hand to pass the needle tip just into the skin.
- Slide the guide tube off the needle, which will now hold in the skin without support.
- Pick up the needle handle between your thumb and forefinger and, with a gentle twist, advance the needle into the skin perpendicularly.

Now ask your subject to repeat the process on your LI4 so you can experience the sensation for yourself. Patients often ask if you have ever had acupuncture.

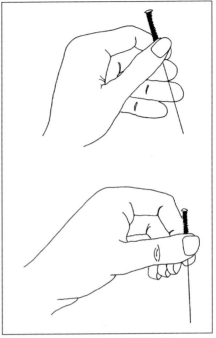

FIG. 2. TECHNIQUE OF NEEDLE GRIP AND MANIPULATION

NB Most needles can be advanced 0.5 to 1 cun depth into the skin. However, always be aware of underlying structures that could be irritated or damaged (e.g. pneumothorax with GB21 or medulla oblongata with GV15). Deep penetration is not essential to achieve good results. Be slow and gentle while advancing a needle. Acupuncture should be as painless as possible to ensure patient compliance. Resting the forearm or wrist on the patient, while advancing a needle with that hand, will help to prevent buried or broken needles if the patient jumps or moves unexpectedly.

To stimulate a needle, gently rotate it back and forth between the thumb and forefinger. This can be associated with gently lifting and thrusting the needle at the same time. Another method is to insert the needle and then gently tweak, or flick it, from side to side with your finger. This often produces a more gentle, more acceptable form of energy transmission through the needle.

Needles can just be inserted, left for twenty minutes and removed. However stimulating the needle to achieve *De-Chi* is probably more effective. De-Chi is the term used to describe a numb or painful sensation around the area of needle insertion that frequently travels along the meridian, either proximally or distally. Once this has been achieved no further stimulation is required and the needle can be removed. The acupuncturist can often feel the tissues tightening around the needle just prior to this point and can stop stimulating. This avoids unpleasant sensations for the patient.

Sometimes when an attempt is made to remove a needle the tissues have grasped it tight and it cannot be removed. Very gentle stimulation of the needle may free it, or conversely, insert another needle adjacent to it and stimulate the second needle slowly until the first is released. Then remove both needles. Dispose of all used needles in standard medical sharps containers.

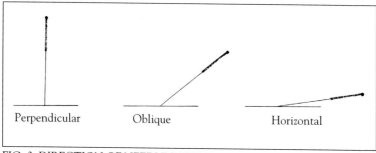

Perpendicular   Oblique   Horizontal

FIG. 3. DIRECTION OF NEEDLE INSERTION

Periosteal pecking is a method of using an acupuncture needle to achieve strong stimulation. It is useful in severe or acute pain. It involves inserting the needle down to underlying bone and gently tapping the point of the needle repeatedly into the periosteum (a bit like a woodpecker action).

Examples of points where periosteal pecking can be useful are CV17 onto the sternum for angina; Ah-Shi points (tender trigger points) overlying the sacrum and sacroiliac joints for low back pain; and GB20 onto the occiput for facial pain. The first few taps are painless but gradually the periosteum starts to register pain and the patient finds it uncomfortable. This is a good time to stop.

COMPLICATIONS

These are few and far between and can be avoided with common sense.

- **Pain on insertion.** Be gentle at all times and try to ensure the patient is as relaxed as possible.

- **Bleeding on removal.** Minimal pressure over the needle site with a sterile swab will stop this. Avoid obvious veins and reassure patients about the benign nature of any resulting bruises at acupuncture sites.

- **Fainting.** More common in anxious patients so encourage them to relax. Treat in the recumbent position rather than sitting. Fainting can be a sign of over stimulation. **For a first treatment do not exceed three needles.** If treating in the sitting position watch closely. If fainting does occur remove all needles immediately, move to the recumbent position and monitor the patient's ABC (airway, breathing and circulation). Reassure the patient that in these situations the acupuncture is invariably very effective.

- **Forgotten needle**. Not uncommon in a busy clinic but rarely a problem for the patient to remove.
- **Infection**. Rarely seen, but always maintain aseptic technique. Infection is more common with press needles in auriculotherapy.

For further information read:

Rosted Palle, 1996, Literature survey of reported adverse effects associated with acupuncture treatment, *American Journal of Acupuncture*, vol. 24, no.1, pp. 27–34.

CONTRAINDICATIONS

The following areas are prohibited for acupuncture:
- Fontanelles
- Breast tissue and nipples
- Umbilicus
- External genitalia

Acupuncture does not cure cancer or malignant disease. However it is very useful for suppressing some of the associated symptoms and syndromes (e.g. pain, depression, insomnia).

Acupuncture should be avoided where there are clear indications for urgent surgery (e.g. acute abdominal pain with peritonism). However, while awaiting a joint replacement, osteoarthritic pain settles well with acupuncture.

The correct treatment of bacterial infection is an appropriate antibiotic, although acupuncture can be complementary by enhancing immunity.

To avoid premature labour or miscarriage refrain from using certain points or strong stimulation during pregnancy. The points to avoid are LI4, SP6 and auriculotherapy.

Conversely these points are useful for induction of labour and pain relief during delivery.

Patients with a tendency to bleed should be needled cautiously and each case should be judged on its merits. Non-invasive stimulation such as acupressure or laser therapy may be more appropriate.

For further information read:

Jayasuriya A, *Clinical Acupuncture*, 11th edn, Sri Lanka, Medicina Alternativa International, pp. 71–89.

RESPONSE TO ACUPUNCTURE: STRONG AND WEAK REACTORS

Initially I achieved a useful response from acupuncture in approximately 60 percent of cases but this increased with experience and further knowledge.

Take note of patients who, on examination, are very tender in the acupuncture points. These people will be strong reactors; they will require fewer needles, less stimulation and fewer treatments.

Patients with no tenderness are likely to be weaker reactors; generally requiring greater stimulation and more treatments.

If there is a large, diffuse area of pain or problematic condition then begin with distal needles and move more proximally with each treatment as the condition settles. Rushing into the painful area may cause a lot of pain during and after treatment. If there is a point area of tenderness or pain then treat with local or Ah-Shi points first.

Most patients have few adverse effects after their treatment. Some say they are worse for twenty-four hours before they improve and others say they feel tired after treatments and need a siesta later that day. I always advise patients to rest for twenty minutes following a treatment as I feel this promotes better results.

In acute conditions treat as often as required to relieve the symptoms, gradually increasing the interval between treatments. Don't treat asymptomatic patients until their problem recurs. One treatment may be curative. In chronic conditions one treatment every one to two weeks is sufficient.

I have recently seen two patients with acute low back pain, both of whom responded immediately to acupuncture to the Ah-Shi points in their quadratus lumborum muscles. In both cases one treatment effected a cure. However another patient, referred by the local pain clinic, with a thoracic strain and twelve months of pain, required multiple treatments spaced two weeks apart. She was not cured, but her visual analogue pain scale* reduced from 8/10 to 3/10 and she was able to reduce from pethidine to simple analgesia.

*For more information on visual analogue pain scales read:

Schneideman I, 1988, Medical Acupuncture: Acupuncture and the Inner Healer, Mayfair Medical Supplies Ltd, Hong Kong, pp. 191–193.

Acute condition: <3/12 duration
Chronic condition: >3/12 duration

Always try to document progress, especially in chronic illness. For example use photographs for skin problems such as psoriasis; or visual analogue pain scores in painful conditions. Without such documentation it can be easy to lose your way.

Most patients should recognise an improvement in their condition in the two weeks following their third treatment. If they do not it is probably not worth continuing with their acupuncture.

When treating chronic conditions that are slow to resolve always consider depression as a possibility and add a sedative series of points.

Children are invariably strong reactors. They only require small needles; minimal stimulation and often at only one acupuncture point. Response to a single 'in / out' needle is often dramatic. Otherwise the same rules of point selection and therapeutics hold for children as adults.

CHAPTER THREE

THE ESSENTIAL ACUPUNCTURE POINTS

There are thirty points that you need to be able to locate and use to start practising acupuncture. I suggest that with each new patient you see you examine for tenderness at these points, even if you don't immediately start treating them. Try and learn the location of a new point each day.

> The descriptions I give will put you in the right location but feel around for **changes in tissue texture, slight depressions or tenderness.** These often give away the exact location.

NOMENCLATURE

The points are named according to which meridian they lie on. For example, there are 67 on the Bladder Meridian, labelled BL1 to BL67. However, you won't need to know all 67.

THE FOURTEEN MERIDIANS

Lung	LU	Kidney	KI
Large Intestine	LI	Pericardium	PC
Stomach	ST	Triple Energiser	TE
Spleen	SP	Gall Bladder	GB
Heart	HT	Liver	LR
Small Intestine	SI	Governing Vessel	GV
Bladder	BL	Conception Vessel	CV

MEASUREMENTS

For measuring distances on the surface of the body (in order to locate points) the unit of measurement is the body inch or CUN. This unit varies according to the stature or size of the patient. It does not relate to the examiner's hand but to the size taken from the patient's hand.

Always check the patient's measurements against your own to evaluate one cun. This will be the width of the patient's thumb or the distance between the interphallangeal joints of the middle finger. Three cun is equal to the width of four of the patient's fingers on one hand. (See fig. 4).

One FEN is one-tenth of a cun. (Fen = 0.1 cun).

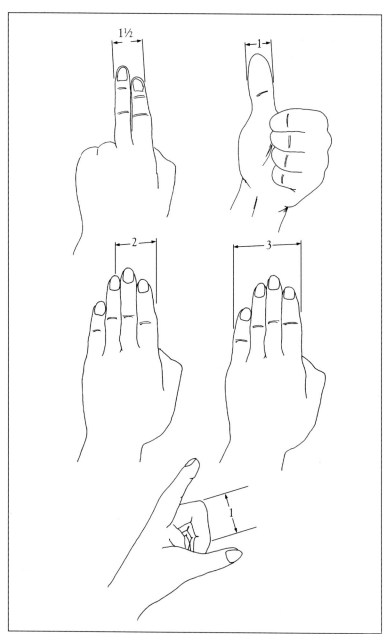

FIG. 4. CUN MEASUREMENTS

POINT DESCRIPTIONS, ILLUSTRATIONS AND PHOTOGRAPHS

Lung

LU7	
Location:	Feel for a groove in the radius, 1.5 cun proximal to the (distal) wrist crease, on the lateral aspect of the forearm.
Indications:	Lung, respiratory and skin diseases
	Has an area of influence over the neck and upper spine

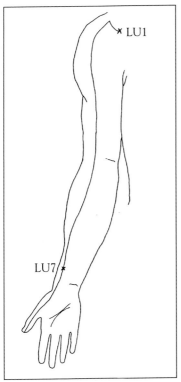

FIG. 5. LUNG
MERIDIAN

Large Intestine

LI4	
Location:	On the summit of the mound created in the first web space by adduction of the thumb. Level with the mid-point of the second metacarpal.
Indications:	Powerful analgesic point
	Has an area of influence over the head and face
	Problems of the wrist and hand
	Disorders and diseases of the large intestine, lungs and skin

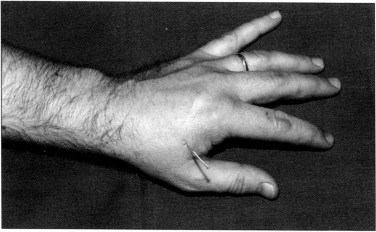

4. LI 4

LI11	
Location:	At the lateral extreme of the antecubital elbow crease when the elbow is semi-flexed.
Indications:	Powerful homeostatic point (e.g. hypertension)
	Problems of the elbow (e.g. tennis elbow)
	Diseases of the lungs (especially involving cough) and skin

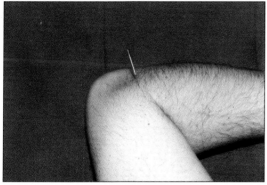

5. LI 11

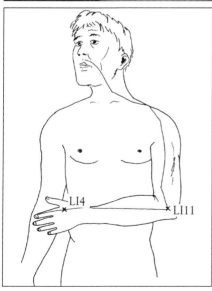

FIG. 6. LARGE INTESTINE
MERIDIAN

Stomach

ST25	
Location:	2 cun lateral to the umbilicus.
Indications:	The alarm point of the large intestine
	Tender and effective in disorders of the large intestine (e.g. constipation, colitis)

ST36	
Location:	0.5 cun (or one finger-breadth) lateral to the patellar tendon insertion, at the level of the inferior tip of the tibial tuberosity.
Indications:	An analgesic and homeostatic point for the lower half of the body
	Has an area of influence over the abdomen
	Effective in gastrointestinal disorders and diseases
	Paralysis of the lower limb
	An immune-enhancing point
	Recommended for mania and psychosis

ST36 is a great point. For an excellent historical summary of the usage of this point and general insight into the history of acupuncture read:

McDonald J, 1996, A short history of point usage: Zusanli,* *Pacific Journal of Oriental Medicine*, no. 6, pp. 35–44.

*Zusanli is the Chinese name for ST36.

ST44

Location:	Just proximal to the web margin between the second and third toes.
Indications:	Excellent analgesic point for the face on the same side (e.g. toothache, trigeminal neuralgia or migraine)

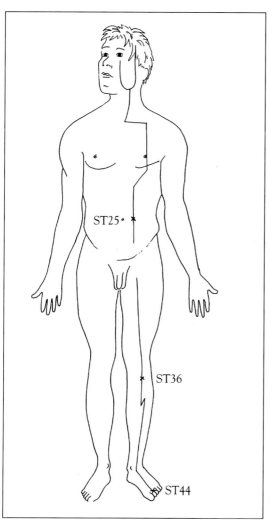

FIG. 7. STOMACH
MERIDIAN

Spleen

SP6	
Location:	3 cun above the inferior margin of the medial malleolus of the ankle on the posterior border of the tibia.
Indications:	Special area of influence over the pelvis and genito-urinary organs
	Obsessive-compulsive disorders
	All conditions with an immunological basis
	General tonification point
	A very powerful point as all the three yin meridians (LR,SP,KI) of the leg cross this point

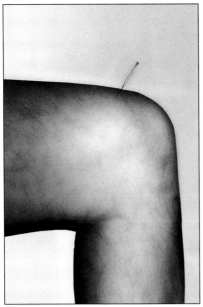

6. SP 10

SP10	
Location:	2 cun above the medial end of the upper border of the patella, on the highest point of the vastus medialis muscle. When examining for this point the patient should be sitting and the knee flexed to 90 degrees.
Indications:	Specific point for itch
	Useful in conditions of the knee

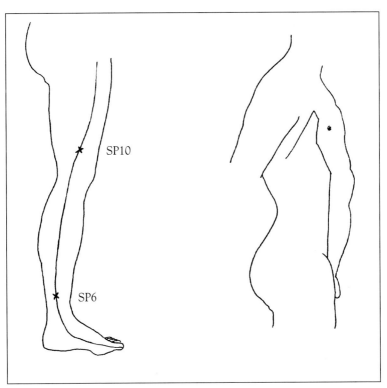

FIG. 8. SPLEEN MERIDIAN

Small Intestine

SI3	
Location:	On the medial end of the transverse crease of the palm of the hand at the neck of the fifth metacarpal. This is most easily found with the hand in a loose fist.
Indications:	Painful conditions of the neck and occiput
	Ear disorders
	In conjunction with its confluent point BL62 it provides good sedation

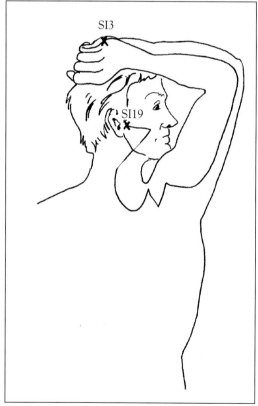

FIG. 9. SMALL INTESTINE MERIDIAN

SI19	
Location:	In the depression created just in front of the tragus of the ear when the mouth is slightly open.
Indications:	All diseases and disorders of the ear
	Temporo mandibular joint (TMJ) problems
	Trigeminal neuralgia

NB This point is usually treated with two other points in front of the tragus (i.e. **TE21** and **GB2**) by using just one needle passed under the skin directly inferiorly from TE21 to GB2.

Heart

HT7	
Location:	On the distal wrist crease, on the radial side of the flexor carpi ulnaris tendon.
Indications:	A powerful sedative point, useful in many psychological and psychiatric problems including anxiety and depression
	Useful in cardiac conditions such as angina and arrhythmia

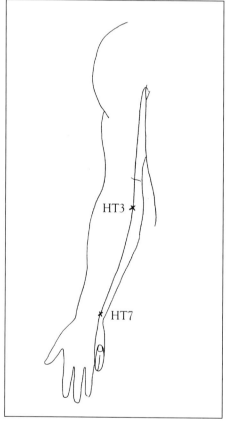

FIG. 10. HEART MERIDIAN

Bladder

BL2	
Location:	In the eyebrow directly above the inner canthus of the eye.
Indications:	Eye disorders
	Frontal sinusitis
	Facial pain
	Low back pain

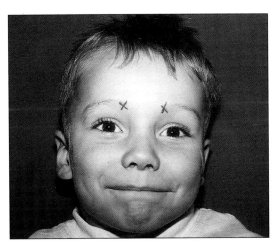

7. BL 2

BL11	
Location:	1.5 cun lateral to the inferior tip of the spinous process of T1.
	NB Angle the needle obliquely towards the vertebra to avoid pneumothorax.
Indications:	An influential point for bones and joints
	Neck and shoulder pain

37

BL40	
Location:	In the mid-point of the transverse popliteal crease.
Indications:	Has an area of influence over the lower half of the back of the trunk
	Low back pain and sciatica
	Knee problems (e.g. Baker's Cyst)

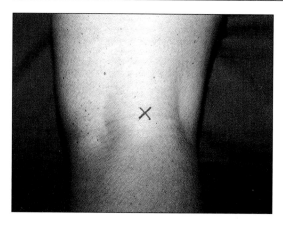

8. BL 40

BL60	
Location:	At the level of the malleolar prominence, mid-way between the lateral malleolus and the Achilles tendon at the ankle.
Indications:	Thoracic spine dysfunction / pain
	Ankle problems
	Achilles tendonitis

BL62	
Location:	In the depression one finger-breadth below the tip of the lateral malleolus of the ankle.
Indications:	Confluent point with **SI3** producing good sedation
	Influential point of the nervous system
	All diseases of the nervous system (e.g. epilepsy, multiple sclerosis)
	Psychological and psychiatric conditions
	Important point for neck pain—'the whiplash point'

NB BL40 is a good distal point for the lower spine; BL60 for the middle and BL62 for the upper spine.

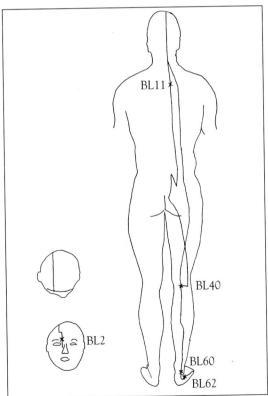

BL11

BL40

BL2

BL60

BL62

FIG. 11. BLADDER
MERIDIAN

Kidney

KI3	
Location:	Opposite BL60 on the medial side of the ankle and can be treated point-to-point with one needle mid-way between the inferior tip of the medial malleolus and the Achilles tendon.
Indications:	Genito-urinary disorders (in combination with SP6)
	Ankle problems

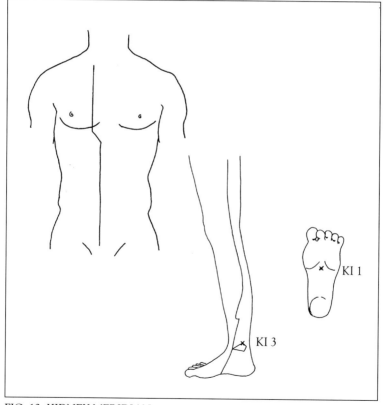

FIG. 12. KIDNEY MERIDIAN

Pericardium

PC6	
Location:	2 cun proximal to the mid-point of the distal wrist crease between the tendons of palmaris longus and flexor carpi radialis. There is often a small, superficial vein crossing the tendons at this point.
Indications:	Nausea. Excellent anti-emetic point
	Area of influence over the chest
	Hyperemesis gravidum
	Often used in combination with **HT7** and for the same indications

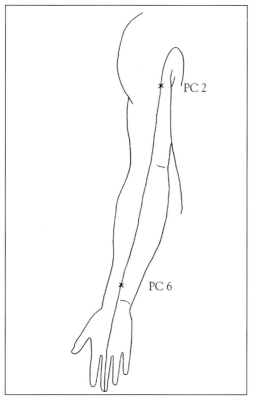

FIG. 13. PERICARDIUM
MERIDIAN

KI

&

PC

Triple Energiser

TE5	
Location:	Opposite PC6 on the dorsum of the forearm and can be treated point-to-point with one needle (i.e. 2 cun above the distal wrist crease between the radius and ulna).
Indications:	Good distal point for ear disorders
	Shoulder disorders
	Works well for muscular and tendon problems when used in combination with **GB34**

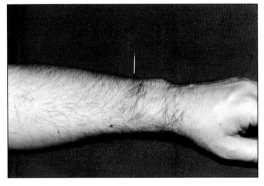

9. TE 5

TE21	
Location:	In the depression just anterior to the supra-tragic notch, with the mouth slightly open.
Indications:	See **SI19**
	Also used in schizophrenia

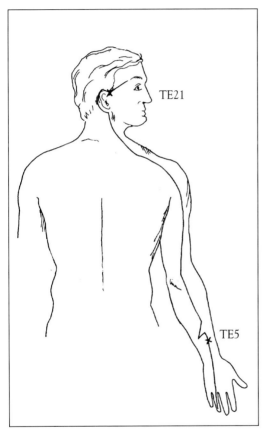

FIG. 14. TRIPLE
ENERGISER
MERIDIAN

Gallbladder

GB2	
Location:	Just anterior to the infra-tragic notch immediately below SI19.
Indications:	See **SI19**

NB An aid to memory for the three points of the ear are (from superior to inferior):

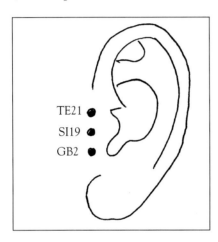

TE21: Top Floor

SI19: Second Floor

GB2: Ground Floor

21–19=2

FIG. 15. GB2 POINT

GB20	
Location:	High in the postero-lateral aspect of the neck, just beneath the occiput. At the apex of the triangle formed by the sternocleidomastoid and trapezius muscles.
Indications:	A good distal point for the face
	Migraine
	Eye and sinus problems
	Neckache and occipital headache

GB21	
Location:	Mid-way between GV14 and the acromio-clavicular (AC) joint of the shoulder, on the upper border of the trapezius. Invariably tender.
Indications:	Neck and shoulder problems, especially where trapezius is implicated

CAUTION: Deep penetration of this point may precipitate pneumothorax. Do not penetrate greater than 0.5 cun.

GB30	
Location:	One-third of the distance on a straight line drawn from the greater trochanter of the femur to the sacral hiatus (or at the junction of the lateral third and medial two-thirds of a line drawn from the greater trochanter of the femur to the sacral hiatus). This point is best located with the patient lying in the lateral or prone position.
Indications:	Hip dysfunction and pain
	Acute sciatica. Requires a long needle with deep penetration over the sciatic nerve (paraesthesia is often elicited on insertion to 5 cun)

GB34	
Location:	Just antero-inferior to the head of the fibula.
Indications:	Influential point for muscles and tendons
	Useful in all soft tissue conditions and injury
	Knee dysfunction and pain
	Diseases of the gallbladder
	Paralysis of the leg

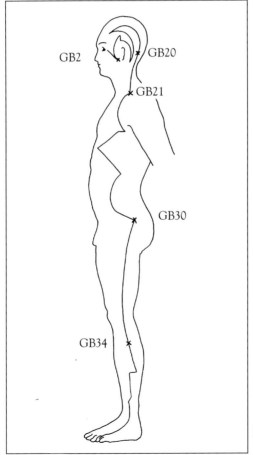

FIG. 16. GALLBLADDER
MERIDIAN

Liver

LR3	
Location:	On the dorsum of the foot, in the depression between the bases of the first and second metatarsals.
Indications:	The most powerful homeostatic point
	Headache and migraine
	Hypertension
	Atopy
	Nausea
	Hyperemesis gravidum

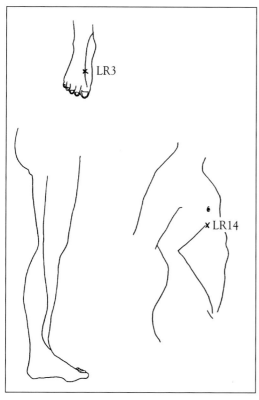

FIG. 17. LIVER
MERIDIAN

Governing Vessel

GV14	
Location:	In the interspinous space beneath C7. (Remember C6 dorsal spine moves away from the examining finger when the patient extends the neck. C7 is then the next dorsal spine below this). An especially strong point, as the three yang meridians of the upper arm pass through it (i.e. LI, SI, TE).
Indications:	Immune enhancement
	Especially good for febrile illness
	Neck and shoulder disorders

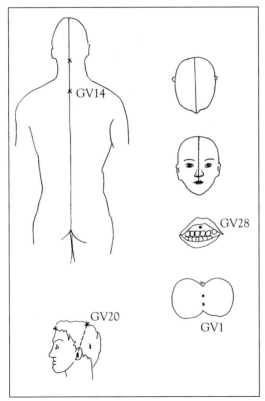

FIG. 18a.
GOVERNING
VESSEL MERIDIAN

GV15	
Location:	0.5 cun above the hairline, in the mid-line between the dorsal spines of the first and second cervical vertebrae. This point is best located with the neck flexed.
Indications:	Strong sedative point and useful in all psychological and psychiatric conditions.
	Speech difficulties following paralytic strokes

CAUTION: DANGEROUS POINT. Do not penetrate more than 1 cun. This avoids damage to the medulla oblongata.

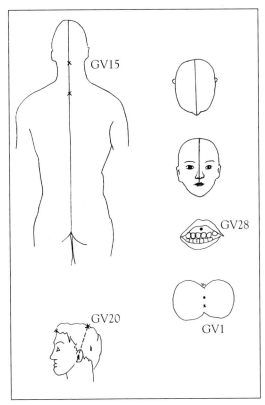

FIG. 18b.
GOVERNING
VESSEL MERIDIAN

Conception Vessel

CV17

Location:	Over the mid-point of the sternum at the level of the nipples (i.e. at the level of the fourth intercostal space).
Indications:	The influential point of the respiratory system
	All respiratory disorders and infections
	Alarm point of the pericardium and therefore all heart disease (e.g. angina)
	Costochondritis

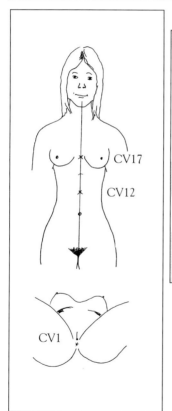

CV12

Location:	4 cun above the umbilicus in the mid-line (mid-way between the xiphoid process and the umbilicus). Penetrate 1.5 cun perpendicularly.
Indications:	Influential point for the Fu (hollow) organs
	Alarm point of the stomach
	An essential point in treating gastrointestinal problems

FIG. 19. CONCEPTION VESSEL MERIDIAN

50

The following photographs are provided to help you revise, and to further illustrate point locations.

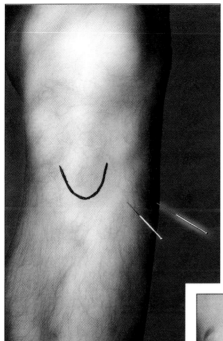

10. ST 36 anterior;
    GB 34 posterior

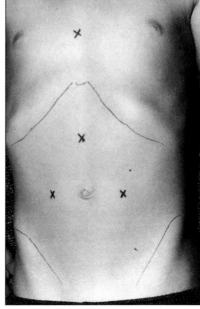

11. CV 17 above; CV 12 middle;
    ST 25 below

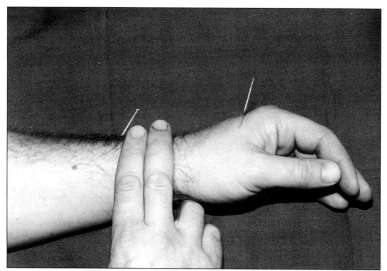

12. LI 4 distal; LU 7 proximal

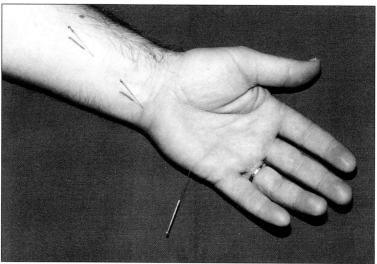

13. SI 3 distal; HT 7 middle; PC 6 proximal

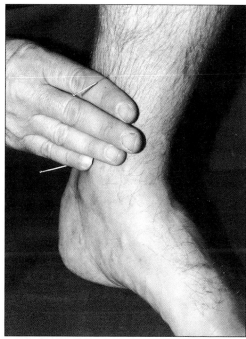

14. SP 6 above; KI 3 below
(separated by 3 cun)

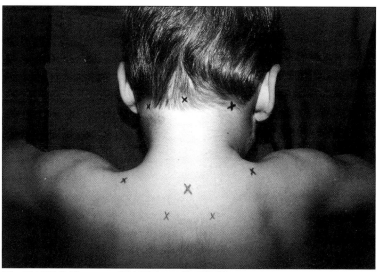

15. HAIRLINE: centre GV 15; laterally GB 20
     NECK: midline GV 14; laterally GB 21; inferiorly BL 11

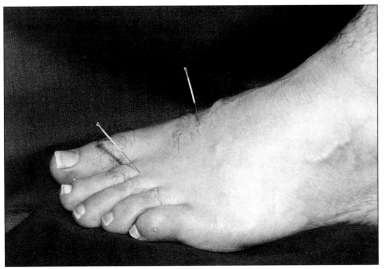

16. ST 44 distal; LR 3 proximal

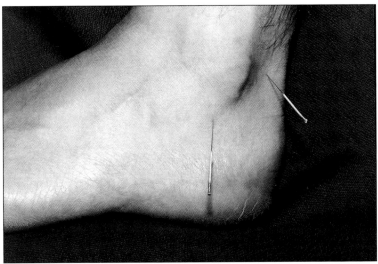

17. LATERAL MALLEOLUS/ANKLE: BL 60 above; BL 62 below

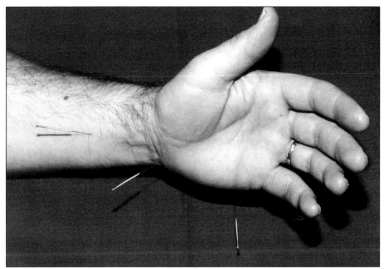

18. SI 3 distal; HT 7 middle; PC 6 proximal

CHAPTER FOUR

THE PRINCIPLES OF POINT SELECTION

1. MERIDIAN POINTS (LOCAL AND DISTAL)

Choose a meridian / channel that overlies the problem area and then treat a point on the meridian both close to the problem (local) and distant from the problem (distal).

For example, in golfer's elbow (lateral epicondylitis) treat LI11 (local) and LI4 (distal). For vertigo (inner ear dysfunction) treat SI19 (local) and SI3 (distal). For a neck problem where trapezius is implicated treat BL11 (local) and BL62 (distal).

2. THE SIX AREA OF INFLUENCE POINTS

There are six area of influence points, three on the arm and three on the leg. Each has a particular area of the body that it is useful for (see fig. 20).

LI4	**Head and face** (e.g. sinusitis, facial pain, toothache, headache)
LU7	**Neck and upper half of the back** (e.g. neck and thoracic back pain)
PC6	**Front of the chest** (e.g. angina, palpitations, intercostal neuralgia, mastitis)
ST36	**Abdomen** (e.g. all pelvic and abdominal problems)
SP6	**Pelvis** (e.g. problems of the external genitalia and all genito-urinary organs)
BL40	**Lower half of the back** (e.g. low back pain, ureteric colic)

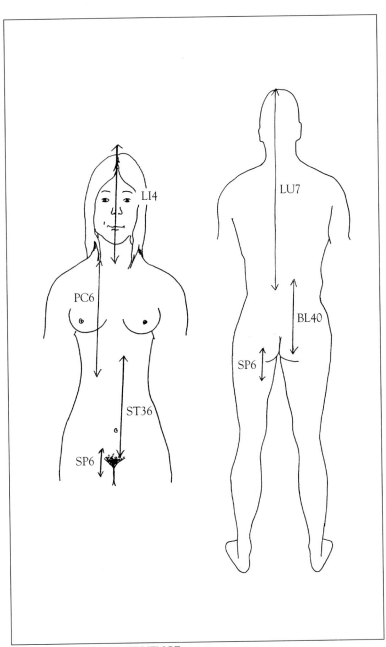

FIG. 20. AREAS OF INFLUENCE

3. ADJACENT LOCAL POINTS

These are points on an adjacent meridian, local to the problem.

For example, with arthritic knee pain you might use ST36, GB34, SP10 and BL40. For a wrist problem consider LU7, LI4, HT7, PC6, TE5 and SI3.

4. AH-SHI POINTS

These are tender points that commonly correspond to the motor points of muscles. If you find a tender point treat it. However, beware of underlying structures.

For example, lumbar paraspinal muscles or quadratus lumborum commonly have Ah-Shi points in low back pain, as do the gluteal muscles. Palpate muscles with first gentle and then more firm pressure. If the patient twitches or complains then you are in the right place. A lot of musculo-skeletal pain can be relieved by treating Ah-Shi points alone or in combination with GB34 and another distal or area of influence point.

5. INFLUENTIAL POINTS

I have listed five commonly used influential points. These have a special influence over specific organs and systems of the body, helping to correct pathophysiology:

CV17	Respiratory disorders
BL11	Bone and joint problems
CV12	Disorders affecting the Fu (hollow) organs (gastrointestinal, bladder, gallbladder etc.)
GB34	Muscle, tendon and injury problems
BL62	Nervous system dysfunction

CHAPTER FIVE

In this section I hope to guide you through the development of prescriptions of acupuncture points that can be adapted to all situations by following the principles of point selection in chapter four. Where I have shown more than one indication for a point then it will be very important in the treatment of that condition (e.g. LI4 is a distal meridian point, area of influence point and a good analgesic point for sinusitis).

MUSCULO-SKELETAL DYSFUNCTION AND PAIN

Generalised conditions, such as polyarthropathy or fibromyalgia may require general points to begin with and then a more focused approach with the more resistant areas. For all painful conditions think LI4; for all injuries and soft tissue problems GB34; and for all joint problems BL11.

Remember when treating points on the back to always aim the needle at the spine by entering the skin obliquely.

Neck	
Meridian Points	
local	GB20, GB21, GV14, GV15
distal	GB34, BL62, SI3
Area of Influence Point	LU7
Ah-Shi Points	Commonly in paraspinal muscles, trapezius, scalenes and sternocleidomastoid
Influential Points	GB34, BL11

Case Study

A patient who had sustained a neck injury as a result of a fall attended the Accident and Emergency Department where I was working as a medical officer. He had pain in the lower neck radiating to the left shoulder for two days. He had also been experiencing some paraesthesia in the left upper arm and elbow. Examination revealed stiffness and pain on neck extension with exacerbation of the paraesthesia. Tone, power and reflexes in the arms were normal. Cervical spine x-ray was normal. Palpation of his neck muscles revealed a tender point in the upper border of his left trapezius at GB21.

Presuming this to be a simple trapezius strain I offered him acupuncture. Despite never having had acupuncture before he was keen to accept. His left GB34 was only minimally tender but as a good distal meridian point and influential point for muscles I elected to treat this first. Since it was not a very tender point I decided to stimulate it quite strongly in the hope of achieving De-Chi (expecting the patient to be a weak reactor). The patient seemed fine initially but then went quite pale and admitted to feeling nauseous and faint. I immediately removed the needle. He was sitting on the edge of the examination bed so I asked him to lie supine for a few minutes until he recovered. I explained that this response to acupuncture was not uncommon and was invariably followed by an excellent result. On rising from the bed the patient's neck was pain-free and fully mobile and his paraesthesia had settled—with just one needle at GB34.

Thoracic Spine	
Meridian Points	
local	BL11, GV14
distal	BL60, BL2
Area of Influence Point	LU7
Ah-Shi Points	These will lie on the BL meridian, 1.5 cun lateral to the inferior aspect of the thoracic, dorsal spines, bilaterally
Influential Points	GB34, BL11

Lumbosacral Spine	
Meridian Points	
local	cf. Ah-Shi
distal	BL40, BL2
Area of Influence Point	BL40
Adjacent Local Point	GB30
Ah-Shi Points	Always palpate the BL points 1.5 and 3 cun lateral to the inferior aspect of the dorsal spines respectively. Three cun lateral will often produce tender points in the quadratus lumborum muscle. Palpate the depressions overlying both sacroiliac joints and treat these with periosteal pecking if tender. The gluteal muscles are commonly in need of treatment
Influential Points	GB34, BL11

This simple approach to low back pain can be a great way to get started in acupuncture.

Case Study

I was doing a locum for a neighbouring GP on the south coast of New Zealand, when a fisherman was helped in by his mates. He had jumped from the dock into his boat and landed awkwardly, twisting his lower back. Initially this had only caused minor discomfort but then he got a severe left lumbar pain on lifting a heavy drum on the deck. He was bent over and unable to straighten his lower back. He felt weak, nauseous and unable to weight bear on the left leg. He was unable to climb onto the examination couch. Examination revealed normal tone, power, reflexes and plantars in the lower limbs. He was excruciatingly tender in the left quadratus lumborum muscle, 3 cun from the mid-line (an Ah-Shi point in the BL meridian). I offered him acupuncture as the most likely treatment to work quickly. I started by treating his left GB34 with strong stimulation to

De-Chi. Then I did the same to both left and right LI4. At this point I waited a few minutes. He was able to stand alone now and I helped him onto the examination couch where he lay in the prone position with chest over a pillow and feet just off the end of the bed. (It is important to have the pillow, not the patient's arms, supporting the patient's weight). His left BL40 was tender and required minimal stimulation to achieve De-Chi. He was still very tender in the Ah-Shi point in the left quadratus lumborum so I elected to insert a needle obliquely here and stimulate it very gently. Insertion was slightly painful but gentle stimulation eased the discomfort and as the tissues tightened around the needle I removed it. Again I let the patient rest for five minutes and then invited him to get up and get dressed. He got off the bed with relative ease and was able to dress with minimal assistance. He was now standing erect and walked out of the surgery in a much more dignified state than when he arrived. I happened to meet him in Queens Park, Invercargill a few days later and he said he had improved steadily after he saw me and was back at work on his fishing boat.

Not all patients respond so dramatically. Advice to return in a few days if the pain recurs or if there has been little response is best. Most patients with acute spinal dysfunction will settle within four weeks with four-to-six treatments. Chronic pain is different and requires fortnightly treatments, often for some weeks or months. Success may be viewed in terms of reduced analgesia or improved depression-rating scores, rather than a complete cure. However don't under-rate the importance of your treatment and supportive doctor-patient relationship in these circumstances. At each visit keep a record of the patient's visual-analogue pain score and drug consumption (prescribed and otherwise), to document improvement.

Sciatica	
	Sciatica should resolve within 12 weeks with acupuncture. If it does not then referral to an orthopaedic surgeon is appropriate for consideration of spinal decompression. GB30, BL40, BL60, BL62 and Ah Shi points in the buttocks are helpful.

Hip Joint	
Meridian Points	
local	GB30
distal	GB34
Area of Influence Point	BL40
Ah-Shi Points	Arthropathy / arthralgia of the hip joint is often associated with tender points in gluteus minimus, tensor fascilata and the adductors of the inner thigh (especially when pain is referred to the knee)
Influential Points	GB34, BL11

This is a great treatment to control arthritic hip pain while a patient is waiting for total hip replacement or if the patient is a poor surgical risk. In the elderly it often avoids the need for non-steroidal anti-inflammatories and their inherent side effects. An initial course of treatment will often drop their visual analogue pain scores from, say, 8/10 to 3/10 and this can be maintained with occasional top-up treatments.

Costochondritis	
	Responds well to periosteal pecking of the costochondral joints, but avoid a pneumothorax. Keep a finger either side of the rib to mark its position when inserting and pecking with the needle.

TMJ Dysfunction

Check for Ah-Shi points in the masseter muscle. Treat TE21, SI19 and GB2 with one needle point-to-point.

Ear or Throat Pain

Check the sternocleidomastoids for Ah-Shi points when there is pain despite normal auroscopy and/or pharyngeal examinations.

Shoulder Pain

Check the scalene muscles for Ah-Shi points. Use periosteal pecking of the coracoid process (i.e. LU1). This is especially good for bicipital tendonitis.

Golfer's and Tennis Elbow

Include periosteal pecking of the medial and lateral epicondyles of the humerus respectively.

Foot Pain, Metatarsalgia and Cramp

Always check the full length of medial and lateral gastrocnemei and soleus (BL57) for Ah-Shi points. Always treat LR3.

Toothache, Facial Pain, Neuralgia

LI4 and ST44 with Ah-Shi points in the masseter muscle.

MIGRAINES AND HEADACHES

Most headaches are classified into different groups such as migrainous / non-migrainous; or classical migraine, tension headache, cluster headaches etc.

One important distinction is a life-long history of migraine compared to a headache of recent origin. Most migraineurs have been investigated fully in the past and typically present with visual aura, nausea and unilateral headache. Generally it will be safe to embark on a trial of acupuncture for these people. However, in its severe form migraine may produce a temporary hemiparasthesia or hemiplegia making it difficult to distinguish from a cerebrovascular accident (stroke) and referral to a doctor, and probably a neurologist, would be appropriate before embarking on acupuncture treatment.

Any headache of recent origin should be investigated by a doctor but while awaiting the outcome of further investigation treatment with acupuncture is appropriate. For example, rapid steroid treatment for temporal arteritis may prevent blindness. Therefore beware the unilateral headache with altered vision and jaw claudication.

Acute headache often settles well with one-to-three treatments over a week and then a fortnightly, monthly or even three-monthly treatment will provide good prophylaxis. For acute migraine always pay attention to treating the patient in the reclining position in a darkened, quiet room. Patients on large doses of Ergotamine or opiate-containing medication will respond poorly to acupuncture. Acupuncture should first be used as part of a drug-withdrawal programme from these compounds before progressing with treatment of headache. Consultation with the prescribing physician is advisable.

NB The most important point for all headaches is **LR3**.

Always start with LR3 as this may give resolution with a single needle. Consider other symptomatic points such as

PC6 for nausea, GB20 for visual disturbances and headache, and SP6 for headache associated with menses. Remember, **don't use LI4, SP6 or auriculotherapy for headache in pregnancy as these points are contra-indicated in pregnancy.**

Headache / Migraine	
Meridian Points	
local	BL2, GB20, GV15
distal	BL62, GB34, ST44
Area of Influence	Point LI4
Ah-Shi Points	Check the neck, temporalis and sternocleidomastoid muscles
Influential Points	GB34, BL62
Don't Forget	LR3

Case Study

A patient with a lifelong history of classical migraine asked if acupuncture would be helpful for her. She said she had infrequent attacks but when they came they laid her out for a week at a time. I suggested that at the onset of her next attack she attend the surgery on an urgent basis. A month later she presented one morning with severe right-sided throbbing headache, photophobia, nausea and vomiting. Examination was unremarkable except for a dilated right pupil. I transferred her to a quiet, dark room and laid her supine on the examination bed. I started treatment by inserting a needle at LR3 and stimulating it strongly to achieve De-Chi. I removed the needle and waited five minutes. On reviewing her she claimed to be feeling less nauseous and her headache was less severe. I moved to her right hand and stimulated LI4 strongly as this is a good analgesic point and area of influence point for the head. On achieving De-Chi I removed the needle and gently stimulated PC6 as an anti-emetic point. Again I left her until I had seen another patient and then reviewed her. By now her nausea had settled completely and she had only a dull thud behind the right eye. To finish my treatment I gave her a little periosteal pecking of the occiput at GB20, stopping before it became uncomfortable. On review the following day her headache, photophobia and nausea had settled but she still felt very lethargic. A review of her systems history revealed some nocturia and urgency. Urinalysis showed leukocytes, blood and protein +++ inferring she had a urinary tract infection. A single dose of trimethoprim returned her to her normal self. Her migraines were infrequent and she refused prophylactic acupuncture in favour of urgent acupuncture for any future attacks.

SKIN

Skin conditions often respond dramatically to acupuncture. It is always worth a trial as it may allow a patient to reduce, or stop, potentially toxic medication such as high dose topical steroids or cytotoxics (e.g. methotrexate, cyclosporin). The principles of treatment are the same as before, but from traditional Chinese medicine (TCM) we know that the skin corresponds to the LU and LI meridians. Points with a strong immune basis are helpful (e.g. allergic dermatitis or urticaria), as are sedative points (especially where there is a psychological exacerbation or depression). Auriculotherapy is especially helpful in skin conditions and the LU and LI auriculotherapy points can be added to therapy.

Skin	
Meridian Points	
local	Choose a meridian that traverses the skin lesion
distal	As above
Adjacent Local Points	Choose the points adjacent to the skin lesion
Don't Forget	LU7, LI4, LI11 (TCM, skin) SP6, ST36, GV14 (immune enhancing) GV15, BL62, S13, LI4, HT7, PC6, LR3 (sedative series for depression) SP10 (for itch)
Auriculotherapy	Lung/large intestine areas

For example, if a person has psoriasis of the dorsum of the feet and elbows (extensor aspect) consider:

Meridian Points	
local	LR3, ST44, TE5
distal	LI4, ST36, TE21
Adjacent local points	SP6, LI11

For further information on the correspondences in traditional Chinese medicine read:

Schneideman I, 1998, *Medical Acupuncture: Acupuncture and the Inner Healer*, Mayfair Medical Supplies Ltd, Hong Kong, ch. 8.

For further information on auriculotherapy read:

Jayasuriya A, *Clinical Acupuncture*, 11th edn, Medicina Alternativa International, Sri Lanka, pp. 765–787.

IMMUNE SYSTEM: ALLERGIES AND INFECTION

In allergy and infection treat general immune points (good for fever) and local points for the area involved. Don't, however, insert needles into *acutely* inflamed skin (e.g. cellulitis). **Remember the appropriate treatment for bacterial infection is antibiotic.**

A good example here is to consider treatment for **rhinitis / sinusitis** (either allergy or infection):

Meridian Points	
local	BL2
distal	LI4, LI11, ST 36, ST44, GV14
Area of Influence Point	LI4
Ah-Shi Points	Overlying the malar bone and / or sphenopallatine ganglia
Influential Points	CV17
Immune Points	**SP6, ST36, GV14**
Don't Forget	LU7

RESPIRATORY DISEASE

Mostly this relates to reversible (asthma) and non-reversible airways obstruction or chronic obstructive airway disease (COAD). My experience of treating asthma with acupuncture is positive, with increasing stability of the airways and reduction in medication requirements. In milder cases acupuncture can gradually replace all medication and be used on a 'top up' basis for asthma prophylaxis.

In COAD I believe that patients derive a subjective, if not always objective, improvement from acupuncture therapy and I am using it increasingly as an adjunct to more conventional therapy. For example, it is a nice alternative to antibiotics for bronchitis (invariably viral in origin) and helps to decrease antibiotic over-prescribing and reduce antibiotic resistant organisms.

Respiratory Disease	
Meridian Points	
local	CV17
distal	LU7, ST36, KI3, SP6
Area of Influence Point	PC6
Ah-Shi Points	Coracoid process (LU1) and 1.5 cun lateral to the inferior aspect of the dorsal spine of T3 bilaterally (BL13, Back-Shu point of the lungs*)
Influential Point	CV17
Immune Points	SP6, ST36, GV14
Don't Forget	LI4, LI11, LU7 (TCM Correspondences)

For further information on Back-Shu points read:

Jayasuriya A, *Clinical Acupuncture*, 11th edn, Medicina Alternativa International, Sri Lanka, p. 428.

Case Study

A fifteen-year-old boy visited me complaining of severe morning catarrh for several months, despite multiple medications including steroid nasal spray. He also had asthma that was controlled with twice-daily steroid inhalation. His father was fed up listening to his son clear his throat and blow his nose constantly before going to school in the mornings and hoped acupuncture could relieve his symptoms. The 'final straw' had been that, for the previous three mornings, he had developed epistaxis (nose bleeds) on blowing his nose.

I treated points on the large intestine and lung channels and an immune series. On review a week later he had had no further epistaxis and his catarrh had reduced slightly. After a further four treatments on a fortnightly basis his nose was clear and he had stopped all nasal sprays. After a further two treatments he stopped all medication and six months later, with a monthly treatment, he is asymptomatic and off all medication including his asthma inhalations. I will continue to see him on an intermittent basis when he develops coryza or cough.

VERTIGO (INCLUDING MENIERE'S DISEASE)

Benign postural vertigo and Meniere's exacerbations can resolve rapidly with acupuncture. Acute viral labyrinthitis also responds well and immune points should also be included. Chronic otitis media responds slowly but steadily.

Remember patients complaining of a combination of unilateral deafness, unsteadiness and tinnitus (buzzing in the ear) should be referred on to a physician for further assessment to exclude acoustic neuroma.

Middle and Inner Ear Disease	
Meridian Points	
local	TE21, SI19, GB2 (point-to-point)
distal	TE5, SI3, GB34, GB20, GV14 (all the yang meridians of the upper limbs pass through this point)
Area of Influence Point	LI4
Ah-Shi Points	Sternocleidomastoid and masseter muscles
Influential Points	BL62
Don't Forget	Immune points for infection and/or sedative series for anxiety / depression

GASTROINTESTINAL PROBLEMS (INCLUDING IRRITABLE BOWEL SYNDROME)

It should be born in mind that gastrointestinal disturbances should be fully investigated to establish aetiology and pathology. It is only appropriate to use acupuncture (or any other treatment) once the underlying pathology has been established or while awaiting results of investigation. Change in bowel habit can be symptomatic of serious underlying diseases, from malignancy to gastroenteritis. Irritable bowel is a diagnosis that should only be considered after careful medical evaluation, and appendicitis requires appendicectomy.

However, acupuncture is very effective at treating gastrointestinal problems. A variety of problems that respond to the following regime are irritable bowel syndrome, diarrhoea, constipation, gastroenteritis, dyspepsia and peptic ulcer pain.

Gastrointestinal Problems	
Meridian Points	
local	CV12, CV17, ST25
distal	ST36, SP6, LR3
Area of Influence Point	ST36
Influential Point	CV12
Don't Forget	LI4, PC6

Case Study

I was doing a locum at an urban practice and after treating several patients with acupuncture the practice nurse enquired whether I would be prepared to treat her husband for his irritable bowel syndrome. He had had acupuncture for it many years previously but it had started to recur.

Further discussion with the husband revealed he had been extensively investigated in the past but had not overcome his problem until he tried acupuncture. After just a few treatments he had been 'cured' and only now, after several years, had the problem recurred. He complained of abdominal discomfort with bloating, alternating constipated and diarrhoea stool and incomplete emptying on defaecation.

I started by treating just three points bilaterally to De-Chi (i.e. ST36, CV12 and LI4). He then rested supine for fifteen minutes and I asked him to return in one week. The following week the patient's abdominal discomfort had resolved but his seasonal rhinitis had started. We therefore changed tack and treated immune points . . . but that's another story.

PSYCHIATRY (INCLUDING ADDICTIONS)

Anxiety, depression, insomnia and restless legs all respond to a sedative series. However, supportive counselling and a good doctor / patient relationship enhance the effect. Treating associated physical problems is also important. While psychotic patients should be seen by a psychiatrist, acupuncture may be a useful adjunct in therapy. Remember many psychiatric patients suffer from associated anxiety and depression. Acupuncture is very useful in withdrawal regimes for addiction to drugs (e.g. nicotine) and alcohol. A sedative series and treatment according to symptomatology is required.

Sedative Series:	
	GV15, LR3, HT7, PC6, (SI3, BL62)

Restless Legs (and Cramp):	
	BL57 and Ah-Shi points in gastrocnemei
	Sedative series

Addictions:	
	Sedative series and points related to symptomatology:
	Headache LI4, LR3
	Myalgia GB34
	Nausea PC6, LR3
	Palpitations PC6, HT7, CV17
	Cough LI11, LU7

For further information read:

Toteva and Milanov, 1996, The use of body acupuncture for treatment of alcohol dependence and withdrawal syndrome: A controlled study, *American Journal of Acupuncture*, vol. 24, no.1, pp. 19–25.

CARDIOVASCULAR DISEASE

No one would question that anti-anginal drugs are the mainstay of medical treatment for ischaemic pain. However, acupuncture may help to reduce dosage of drugs and alleviate side effects. For example, less betablocker may mean less lethargy, unpleasant dreams or claudication. Less calcium channel blocker may relieve peripheral oedema and indigestion. Less nitrate means reduced headache. The anxiety and depression associated with cardiac disease is relieved by a sedative series. Innocent palpitations (e.g. controlled atrial fibrillation) may be relieved with acupuncture. Remember, as a general rule, palpitations and arrhythmia should be investigated by a physician. Atypical, non-specific chest pain is often ignored by the medical profession but can respond well to acupuncture.

Hypertension may respond but will require lifelong therapy and a large commitment on behalf of both the acupuncturist and patient. However, it can definitely be a useful adjunct to medical therapy. Never forget the importance of counselling for dietary and smoking habits.

Cardiovascular Problems	
Meridian Points	
local	CV17 (periosteal pecking)
distal	KI3, ST36, HT7, PC6
Area of Influence Point	PC6
Ah-Shi Points	1.5 cun lateral to the inferior aspect of the dorsal spines of T4 and T5, bilaterally. (BL14, BL15, Back-Shu points for the pericardium and heart)*
Don't Forget	LI4 (pain)

For further information on Back-Shu points read:

Jayasuriya A, *Clinical Acupuncture*, 11th edn, Medicina Alternativa International , Sri Lanka, p 428.

GENITO-URINARY PROBLEMS

Renal colic often responds well to acupuncture, avoiding the side effects of opiates or non-steroidal anti-inflammatories. Chronic cystitis and bladder neck disorders as well as mild prostatism will often respond to acupuncture.

Renal / Ureteric Colic	
Meridian Points	
local	cf. Ah-Shi points
distal	BL60, BL40, BL2, SP6
Area of Influence Points	BL40, ST36, SP6
Ah-Shi Points	1.5 cun lateral to the inferior aspect of the dorsal spine of L2, bilaterally (BL23, Back-Shu point of kidney)*
Don't Forget	LI4 (pain)

* For further information on Back-Shu Points read:

Jayasuriya A, *Clinical Acupuncture*, Medicina Alternativa International , 11th edn, Sri Lanka, p. 428.

Case Study

An obese patient in her twenties with fibromyalgia had been having acupuncture predominantly for spinal pain for which I had been using bladder points extensively. At her second visit she admitted she had been having urinary incontinence for many months but that it stopped abruptly on commencing acupuncture. This is attributable to treatment of her bladder meridian. BL60, BL40, BL23 and BL2 are common points for spinal pain.

OBSTETRICS AND GYNAECOLOGY (INCLUDING PRE-MENSTRUAL TENSION)

Acupuncture in obstetrics is limited to cases where the benefit will outweigh the possible risk of miscarriage.

Avoiding the prohibited points in pregnancy is important (i.e. LI4, SP6, auriculotherapy). Remember these points can induce labour or miscarriage. Other miscarriages after acupuncture are likely to be spontaneous but a thorough discussion with the patient outlining risks and possible benefits should be part of the routine of treatment in pregnancy. A signed patient consent form may be appropriate.

Hyperemesis Gravidum responds well to acupuncture, especially PC6 and LR3.

Hyperemesis Gravidum	
Meridian Points	
local	CV12
distal	ST36, **LR3**
Area of Influence Point	ST36
Influential Point	CV12
Don't Forget	**PC6**

Case Study

A patient with a history of hyperemesis in her first pregnancy (requiring multiple hospital admissions for rehydration and anti-emetics) was referred to me six weeks into her second pregnancy because she had started to vomit. She did not like needles but would allow me to use three per session if they were inserted and left unstimulated for thirty minutes and then removed. On each occasion I checked her bilateral points for tenderness at PC6, LR3 and ST36, then I placed one needle at each of these points on the most tender side. I repeated this every second day for three treatments and she started to improve after the second treatment. By eight weeks we were down to a weekly treatment that lasted until twenty weeks when her nausea stopped completely. Until this time she had not been completely free of nausea but she could eat and had no vomiting or admissions to hospital. The patient was very satisfied with this in comparison to her previous experience.

Induction of labour and pain relief for delivery: LI4, SP6 (strong stimulation)

By now you can see that in learning just a very few acupuncture points, a midwife, general practitioner-obstetrician or an obstetrician can provide useful, adjunctive acupuncture therapy for their patients.

In gynaecology many disorders respond well to acupuncture and adding a sedative series for pre-menstrual tension can be extremely beneficial. Other problems that respond well are dysmenorrhoea, menorrhagia, endometriosis and pelvic inflammatory disease.

Gynaecology	
Meridian Points	
local	Sacral foraminae (Bl3 to BL35)
distal	BL40, SP6, LR3, ST36, KI3
Area of Influence Point	SP6
Ah-Shi Points	On the CV meridian in the mid-line between the symphysis pubis and umbilicus (CV2 to CV6)
Influential Point	CV12
Don't Forget	Sedative series for pre-menstrual tension

Case Study

A patient in her early thirties enquired whether acupuncture would be helpful for her endometriosis. Her only relief from dysmenorrhoea was Danazol and although she had been offered another course, she felt unable to tolerate the side effects. She suffered from right iliac fossa pain of grade 9/10 (visual analogue pain score) from the day before her period to the day after (i.e. five days in total). The bleeding was quite heavy and she felt generally unwell and nauseous throughout the period and beyond. I explained that the result was not predictable and that of four people treated with acupuncture two will get a good response (therapeutic), one will get a response that will be helpful (a useful adjunct) and one is not helped by acupuncture — however I was happy to try.

I treated her on alternate days, three times per week, for the week leading up to each period, each time using the gynaecology points outlined above. She noticed very little change during her first period but started to improve during her second period. After her third period she recalled that instead of five miserable days she was suffering only five miserable hours. Her bleeding had settled to a trickle and her nausea and general health had improved dramatically. As a spin off she had also noticed that she had a softer motion that was less likely to become constipated, and that she had recovered from an upper respiratory infection much more promptly than usual. I treated her again but she had slightly more pain than with the previous period. The only difference in treatment was that I had not included Ah-Shi points over her sacral foraminae as before. I included them thereafter.

After five consecutive months / periods I enquired how she was feeling about the treatment. She felt happy to continue with two-to-three treatments in the week before each period for the foreseeable future, at least until she came to a decision about possible hysterectomy. Unfortunately the endometriosis was associated with infertility, making hysterectomy rather unpalatable. Leading on from this the patient asked about fostering children and we had quite a discussion.

 Don't forget there is more to acupuncture
than just sticking needles into people.

REFERENCES AND FURTHER STUDY GUIDE

Useful Sources of All Acupuncture Equipment and Books:

1. Mayfair Medical Supplies Ltd, Kowloon, Hong Kong.

   Tel: ++852 2721 0291   Fax: ++852 2721 2851
   Email: mayfair@hk.super.net

2. Morgan & Aickin, PO Box 13–242, Onehunga, Auckland, New Zealand.

   Tel: Tollfree 0800 656 611.

3. Acu-Needs, 294 Wonga Rd, Warranwood, Victoria 3134, Australia.

Journals:

1. American Journal of Acupuncture, PO Box 610, Capitola, California 95010, USA.

2. New Zealand Journal of Acupuncture, PO Box 164, Lyttelton, New Zealand.

Textbooks:

1. Jayasuriya A, *Clinical Acupuncture*, 11th edn, Medicina Alternativa International, Sri Lanka.

2. Schneideman I, 1988, *Medical Acupuncture: Acupuncture and the Inner Healer*, Mayfair Medical Supplies Ltd, Hong Kong.

3. Helms J M, 1995, *Acupuncture Energetics: A Clinical Approach for Physicians*, Medical Acupuncture Publishers, Berkeley, USA.

Distance Learning Course for Doctors:

Acupuncture (MFM1018),
Graduate Diploma of Family Medicine,
Dept of Community Medicine and General Practice,
Monash University, 867 Centre Rd,
East Bentleigh,
Victoria 3165, Australia.

Tel: ++61 3 9579 3188   Fax: ++61 3 9570 1382.

Acupuncture Courses in Sri Lanka:

Contact: Professor Anton Jayasuriya,
Institute of Acupuncture, Homeopuncture and
Lasertherapy, Colombo South Govt General Hospital,
Kalubowila, Sri Lanka.

Courses and Societies:

1. Medical Acupuncture Society of New Zealand,
   PO Box 164, Lyttelton, New Zealand.

2. Medical Acupuncture Society of Australia,
   PO Box 7930, Bundall, Queensland 4217, Australia.

   Tel: ++61 7 559 26699   Fax: ++61 7 559 26770
   Tollfree: 1800 803853

3. British Medical Acupuncture Society,
   Newton House, Newton Lane, Whitley,
   Warrington, WA4 4JA, UK.

   Tel: ++44 1925 730727   Fax: ++44 1925 730492

   Internet: http://users.aol.com/acubmas.bmas.html